KLAUS KOEPPE

A Mental Medicine Chest

The spiritual causes and significance of desease

A Mental Medicine Chest

By Klaus Koeppe

The spiritual causes and significance of disease

Translated into English by Joyce Nelson-Smith

Overview

Preface

This booklet is a kind of mental medicine chest – nothing more. It is intended for people who have already dealt with this sort of approach to the subject. I do not claim to be scientific nor comprehensive. To start with, I would like to refer to Louise L. Hay who has written a classic book, "Heal Your Body" on the subject of understanding the symptoms of illness and whose writings have taught me the basics. I am not trying to re-invent the wheel, so this little booklet is only meant to expand on the information and interpretation given by Louise Hay. I look upon my contribution as a supplement and not an alternative.

I have written this booklet especially for those who have demonstrated their confidence in me by taking part in my study courses and who may wish to continue to work on themselves. I was not always able to concentrate on everyone individually and I hope that this booklet might help to give one or the other of them the possibility of continuing to work on the healing process.

The aim of this booklet is to encourage you, dear reader, to recognise and feel what is important and consequently to discover your knowledge within yourself. Everything I am writing here is in some way a basic truth and part of our intrinsic human knowledge. Or else it would be nonsense.

I, of course, believe it to be true and that this truth dwells in all of us, because it affects all of us. Just as the fact that we have legs means that we can walk, the fact that we fall ill means that illness has a meaning and that we can all heal ourselves if we wish.

Have confidence that you know everything that you want to know. The connection between disease and spiritual problems is in you, in each one of us. This connection is there whether you believe in it or not. However, if you open up, this knowledge will begin to grow – first through reading, then through experience and finally through yourself. You will see. But first of all you must get involved and give it a go.

There is only one condition for every one of us on this journey of discovery:

Be absolutely honest with yourself!

A scientific world view and the wisdom of life

We live in a world where extensive popular materialism determines the world view of most people. Even those who are deeply religious and believe in God and in life after death find that their ordinary conscious deeds are led by material considerations. Facts dominate us. This has led, I believe, to a frightening number of people losing contact with their innermost feelings. They prefer to give credence to any so-called study rather than their own feelings and inclinations. Every medical practitioner has become a pseudo-god; medicine is expected to produce new wonders all the time. Spiritually, the psychotherapist has become a substitute for a friend. Our readiness to depend on the knowledge and opinion of others, of so-called professionals, has become enormous. In the process, a lot of our natural original knowledge has been lost.

Modern natural sciences dominate our world view and most importantly, they determine how most people in the western world feel about themselves and their circumstances. In the course of this development, disease has become a kind of biochemical interlude where the individual participates only as the victim. The surgeon or the chemistry of the medication are expected to put everything right. Illness has become a "stroke of fate", a mystery that can only be resolved or altered by the doctor or some other professional, because they have studied the matter and know better than the person concerned.
The blind basis for this attitude lies in our subconscious conviction that:

Matter dominates our life and our body
I consider this assumption to be false and misleading.

All my experience and all my knowledge is based on the conviction that the spirit dominates matter. I do not subscribe to the popular idea of a modern material world, determined by the rules of natural sciences. When I speak of the spirit, I do not mean the human

5

intellect, although it is part of the spirit. For me, the notion "spirit" includes all the energies that influence our existence: mental energies, thoughts, feelings – our fears and needs – moods, imagination, attitudes, mental and psychic programmes that we follow all the time, and also spiritual energies including those for which we have no name because we do not know them yet or because we suppress or deny them.

To you, dear reader, it may sound odd that I regard feelings as signs of the existence of the spirit. We all know from experience that strong emotions immediately affect our body so that for instance fear causes us to break out in a sweat, to blush, to tremble etc. The emotions themselves are non-material realities that constantly influence and direct our body without pause.

The world around us suggests that matter and its laws impact upon us and create our illnesses. There are many studies that make genetic influences responsible for our health. Nutrition, environment and genes are the most widely accepted external factors. If you believe this, then this book will be difficult for you to understand, because I believe on the contrary that every person creates his own health or disease. My philosophical standpoint is that the spirit dominates matter. Our spirit therefore puts its stamp on the environment and on all those influences that we wish to admit and finally also on our genes.

In order to gather valuable knowledge about life, we should therefore study the spirit and its laws rather than matter. This is the aspiration of this book. Only by recognising spiritual reality will we be able to regain our old knowledge slumbering within us and waiting to be drawn into the light of our consciousness.
The contents of this booklet will only be of use to you if you accept that this basic tenet is at least possible: spirit dominates matter and therefore also our body.

Responsibility for one's own health or illness

I contend, and I shall justify my opinion, that everybody, without exception, is responsible for his or her own health. We create our illnesses and we also heal ourselves. Doctors support our recovery but we are the ones who do the actual healing.

Yes, you read correctly! I claim that everyone creates his own disease, even those who suffer from cancer or MS or even from accidents. You may wish to dispute this statement or argue that I have made it too boldly.

What is bothering you is possibly mistaking responsibility for blame. People often think that I am saying that sick people only have themselves to blame. I am not, because to blame is to judge or to condemn. I am certainly not judging anyone and certainly not someone who is ill. For me, the notion of health is not a moral one; it is not a question of blame or apportioning blame. It is about understanding the creation of good or bad health and healing.

Responsibility is entirely different from blame. Responsibility has to do with power, and means that I am the cause of an event, quite unconnected with any moral evaluation. Responsibility means that I myself am the response to what has happened or is happening. The response is within me and not outside of me. The reason why the response is within me is because I have created the situation or I was at least deeply involved in it.

If you wish to continue to be the victim of your illness, then this booklet is not for you. You had better put it away.

Its aim is to encourage you and help you to heal yourself.

The structure of the human personality

In order show the effect of the spirit on the body I shall sketch the structure of the human personality, limiting myself to the basic elements. Here again, I lay no claim to being comprehensive.

In broad terms, our innermost, invisible, spiritual and emotional personality is in three parts, similarly to our body. Looking at our body, there are three "floors": the head at the top, the rump or core including the arms and thirdly the legs. Similarly, you can imagine that there are three "spiritual sections" of comparable dimensions: the conscious – corresponding to the head; the subconscious – corresponding to the core; and the unconscious – corresponding to the legs.

1. The conscious

Basis the comparison with the body, the conscious is the smallest section of our personality. This must seem rather odd given that in our everyday life the modern world is defined by our conscious. Modern technology is the result of man's conscious advances in natural sciences too. When we switch on the electricity, use our mobile phones, drive our cars, use the computer, surf the internet, board a flight, manipulate genes and use all kinds of machines – we are utilising the fruits of man's conscious. Although the results of human consciousness have shaped, dominated and defined our lives enormously, the conscious itself is only the smallest part of our whole personality. The conscious does not really have the power that we are inclined to attribute to it. It is basically only an executive organ. The essential impulses come from the subconscious or even deeper down, from the unconscious.

The typical functions of the conscious are: to rationalise, analyse, abstract, organise, compute, compare, control, orientate, generalise, respect or alter rules, recognise similarities etc.

The conscious is our "window on the world" with the duty to inform us and make us able to survive in our environment, and to make us able to adapt and organise our safety in the widest sense. Because this is its function, the conscious is oriented to the outside world and cannot look inwards or only by a circuitous route. Basis our comparison with the body, the eyes would be a good example. Our eyes always only look outwards in a fairly limited angle, but never inwards or behind. The human conscious is similar. This is why we human beings always need another person (you), to get to know ourselves. Self-knowledge without other people is not possible for the human conscious.

Although it is quite unaware of the connection, the conscious is of course always connected to the subconscious, but there is a kind of filter between the two. This filter hinders undesirable information from surfacing and coordinates the flow of information between the conscious and the subconscious. This filter can easily be manipulated for instance through alcohol, drugs fever, sleep deprivation etc. People say that children and drunks speak the truth ("Out of the mouth of babes…" "In vino veritas"). In children the filter is not yet developed and in drunks the filter is leaky. The behaviour of a drunken person shows his "true" character and not the character that he shows in a wakeful and sober state. The conscious does not always show us and others our "true" self, but a controlled and manipulated variant.

This filter differs from person to person and from culture to culture and is the reason why for instance psychotherapeutic healing can take a long time, in fact on average two years! We also use this filter to govern our repressions.

2. The subconscious

Our subconscious contains our mental and psychological "programmes" according to which we "function". This is like our "software" albeit a very emotional package. In this respect, the conscious can be understood as the sector that carries out the programmes stored in the subconscious without actually being aware of doing this.

I speak of "programmes" and "software", but I would like to avoid any misapprehension that their contents are in any way neutral. Quite the contrary: the contents of the subconscious are all highly emotional. Strictly speaking, there is no rationality in the subconscious. This huge sector of our human personality is entirely emotional.

Among the most important **programmes** governing our functions are the **values and standards** internalised and stored in our childhood which shape our conscience. Our **conscience** is neither religious nor supernatural, but it is a sense within us, that ensures that we continue to belong to those people who are important to us. Values and standards are programmed initially in childhood to give us guidelines in our subconscious. Our conscience ensures that we do not offend against these values and standards and that we thus continue to have a bond with those persons or groups whose recognition and acceptance are vital to us. To offend against one's own conscience can lead to grave self punishment and even self induced death. A person or a group with whom we have the strongest inner bond can continue to define our conscience and hence our values and standards and can continue to influence and alter them for a whole life-time. Religious sects and conversions are a good example of this bond. Adults can suddenly change their values and standards in their subconscious and consequently re-programme their conscience, provided always that there is a strong connection with others. Intellectuals and people educated in the humanities in

Germany suddenly became fanatical racists and even mass murderers for the "Fuehrer". At present there is an endless wave of Islamic suicide bombers. Our world gives us many examples of how the subconscious works.

Our subconscious also contains many **fears and needs** that jointly determine our character and personality. Our experiences, our memories and our prejudices (both our own and assimilated ones) are all stored in our subconscious.

Our expectations are also mostly subconscious. They only become conscious when they are not fulfilled and we find ourselves disappointed and must acknowledge that we have deceived ourselves with our subconscious expectations.

Our **conception of the world** is a very important part of our subconscious mind because, basically, we accept it as it is presented to us. As children we do not question our parents' worldview and as adults we adhere to that view of life that gives us the greatest sense of safety. It is precisely because the conception of life is so emotionally charged that thousands and thousands of people have become its victims over the course of history. Ever since the crusades, we have gone to war in the name of our conception of the world. And even without actual war, people are still being murdered because they do not share a specific philosophy of life.

The conception of life is the foundation stone in our subconscious for our sense of mental safety. If our conception of life is shattered, then **EVERYTHING** is at risk, the whole mental and emotional safety structure of the individual, affecting the values and standards governing moral constraints.

The fact that our world view can change shows that the contents of the subconscious are basically subjective programmes, and that they are **BELIEFS.**

When we study the subconscious more deeply, we will find that our view of the world and hence of our whole life is based on beliefs or on convictions that we have accepted and interiorised. The apparent objectivity with which we regard our world and our experiences is dramatically called into question through this discovery, because this discovery means that we have lost our assumed safety.

11

To sum up, I call the strongest and most effective programmes and forces in the subconscious **SETS OF BELIEFS** or belief patterns. Our concept of the world and of our self lies here. These beliefs act like the operating centre and govern all the other sectors of our personality. Our subconscious stores the concept we have of our self, what we really believe about ourselves, about our value or lack of value, about our chances, faults and insufficiencies. These sets of beliefs shape our thinking, our feelings, our actions and of course the resulting experiences we make in everyday life. We actively create our own experiences, albeit not consciously. We create ourselves a world in the shape we believe it to be.

Only the structure of the subconscious is a given, its contents are variable and therefore dependant on the socialisation of the individual person. This means: Everybody has values and standards; everybody therefore has a conscience but it can have very different and often contrary contents. What can be seen as a value by one person may be abhorrent to the next. It is also possible for completely contrary values to exist side by side as, for example, a very religious Mafia Godfather might be a professional murderer and yet recite his Ave Marias and go to church every Sunday with his family to pray.

The subconscious is also in part constituted by language and can therefore be influenced by language. The structure of the subconscious is a given but the contents grow and are dynamic.

3. The unconscious

The "lowest" sector in my imagery represents the unconscious. As the word suggests, this is an area which is not readily accessible to the conscious mind. To my knowledge, the contents of the unconscious can only be reached in three indirect ways: through dreams and their interpretation, through illness and its symbolic understanding, and through hypnosis.

Our **urges** are the most important forces of the unconscious. These are essentially our instinct of self preservation, aggression, sexuality and an instinctive need for comfort and love, and also the death wish.

Urges are natural basic instincts that act like sleeping volcanoes that suddenly erupt when a situation arises and provokes them into action.

As long as we have enough to eat and drink, live in a nice flat and have enough money, our instinct of self-preservation will hardly be active. If however we are in a threatening situation – war, danger to our life – this instinct will click in and we can react with amazing force.

Conversely, the death wish is activated if we are desperately miserable, depressed or extremely sad. For us humans, death is the very last solution to our problems. If a problem is so massively intractable and so menacing that we cannot find another way out, the death wish gives us the strength and energy to kill ourselves, either consciously by suicide or unconsciously through a mortal illness or a fatal accident.

Our **earliest childhood experiences** are also stored in the unconscious. These include emotional impressions and experiences during our mother's pregnancy. As an embryo we intuitively know how our mother feels about us, whether we are wanted or not, and whether our mother is looking forward to having us or whether she thinks we are a burden...

Even further down in the unconscious there are **memories and experiences of earlier lives**. These are generally so deeply buried that very few people are ever consciously in contact with them. Sometimes, in the later part of a person's life there are vague indications of the stored information through some affinities to certain places, countries, cultures, languages races, landscapes...

The unconscious has its own reality which is distinct from the subconscious. Not only is the unconscious governed by urges that are dictated by natural basic instincts, but it also has its own language – the language of symbols and images.

While the subconscious is constituted strongly by words, these are totally lacking in the unconscious.

The power of creation

The subconscious and the unconscious both constantly create experiences without us having any awareness of this process. It happens at various levels and with the help of various channels of energy.

Our conscious mind, or our conscious ego, serves both these other instances. Our mind gives form and turns into reality the information stored in the unconscious and in the subconscious. With the help of our conscious we create for ourselves power, safety, respect, status, recognition etc. All these needs are not part of our conscious mind but of deeper layers. ***Our conscious is an executive organ.*** Our western world is a good example: our civilisation is "governed by the head" which means that it is very considered, very aware, and very abstract. Most of the rest of the world is much more emotional and less abstract and cool. That is why the western world was able to develop astounding technology – as a result of intense scientific research – and with the aim of dominating nature more and more and better and better. The motor of the western European (and U.S.) civilisation is a gigantic power mania, an enormous ego-operated machine which the participants are entirely oblivious of. We have created a highly emotional dynamic which demands that everything should be "higher- faster- larger" and we have become its victims. Our world of humans, the society that we live in, - and under which many are now suffering – has all been created by us humans, it is a human creation. Our conscious has carried out what was programmed at the inner levels. We all often do things consciously although we know full well that they harm us and do not serve life in the long run. But the pressure from within is too strong, so we do not desist nor do we make lasting changes. This is creation with the help of our conscious mind –despite the fact that we know better.

A different kind of creation happens entirely unconsciously. It is driven by our unconscious programmes, our set of beliefs, views and feelings. This creation happens exclusively at an energy level, based on attraction and rejection. Positive thoughts and feelings attract positive experiences. Negative thoughts and feelings attract negative experiences. This unconscious creation is not recognised by most people, or it is even denied and then called chance. With this word, people are shirking their responsibility for their own experiences, their own life – and even for their illness or good health.

The power of repression

A typically human characteristic is to repress disagreeable thoughts, experiences, problems and memories. We push them out of our conscious into the depths of our personality. In principle, we can push them to any level of our personality. Some may lie only just below the surface of our conscious (viz. short-term forgetfulness, misplacing objects etc.). How deeply an issue is "hidden" from the conscious – and repression means hiding – will depend on the degree to which the individual rates the issue as dangerous or uncomfortable. By hiding apparently dangerous feelings, thoughts, desires and problems from our mind, we empower ourselves. The energies of our conscious are thus available to cope with the daily grind and we feel safe.

Repression is not only useful to our conscious but it is a necessary dynamic. No one can keep all his problems and fears in the forefront of his mind without going mad or at least being unable to pursue his daily life

However, the repressed issues are by their essence energies that do not simply cease to exist by being repressed. On the contrary, repression needs strength and energy. Both the conscious and the subconscious have to exert energy constantly in order to maintain the repression. Pressure generates counter-pressure. Thus the repressed issues gain energy by the very fact of their repression and then push to resurface into the conscious. The unconscious has no "drainage" in its depths. The only channel is into and through the conscious. So the repressed issues push "upwards" into the conscious where they need to be worked through in order to drain away.

Understandably, we mainly repress feelings, thoughts, wishes, initiatives and problems that we are afraid of and that seem dangerous or disagreeable.

Having been repressed into the unconscious, these issues develop a dynamic independent existence. They absolutely want to penetrate

15

into the conscious. To achieve this, they use images and symbols, which are the language of the unconscious.

The most usual and simple attempt to rise into the conscious is through dreams. Our conscious mind is switched off in sleep and the repressed issues can now use detours to enter. Although our conscious is switched off, we can experience images and very exciting and emotional stories at night. We are confronted with our repressions, encoded in pictures, stories and symbols.

But our unconscious is not only active at night. It also plies us with symbolic acts when we are awake and tries to speak to the conscious through for example accidents, apparent coincidences, little incidents...

The repression of spiritual issues is the cause of physical illness. The energy of the repressed issues enters the body and creates illness as a result of trying to communicate with the conscious. The energy had to manifest itself in the body because it could not enter the conscious mind.

Illness is the symbolic language
of the unconscious with our conscious.
Illness based on repression can be healed through awareness and
positive change.

This is the central message of this book.

When the repression is removed, the hidden problems, feelings, thoughts and urges are able to become conscious and the body is unburdened and becomes able to heal. This very important first step is however not always enough and a *change* is required which can at times be very radical.

In the following text the reader will recognise similar feelings reappearing as the causes of all our illnesses, connected of course with concrete problems and conflicts. The strongest feelings are: guilt, being victimised, hate, anger, grudges, rage, fear and fear again, humiliation, excessive demands, inferiority complex etc.

The language of symbols

A symbol hides a reality from the conscious. This reality is hidden because it does not appear as itself but intercedes through a different medium. Because the essence of the symbol's reality is hidden, the conscious has no direct access to symbols.

A symbol only works on the unconscious, it communicates directly without detour with the unconscious. **The conscious does not actually deal with symbols, but only with signs**. The conscious is unable to communicate with symbols. As soon as the conscious analyses and "understands" a symbol, it ceases to be a symbol. For the conscious, the essence is "hidden" in a third party, i.e. in the symbol

Examples: The conscious mind sees a ring but cannot relate directly to it. It is just a ring which may imply a relationship but that relationship is not actually present in the ring as far as the conscious is concerned.
The conscious mind sees bread and wine at Communion but it cannot note the presence of Christ but only assume it or take it for granted.

The essence and the meaning are present in the symbol in terms of energy and immediacy. And this is the reality of the symbol – the direct presence of the essence in the non-essence.
Examples: For the unconscious, marriage is directly present in the marriage ring, not only as a sign. A religious example: In Communion, Christ is present as a real energy and can be experienced. The "other" (bread and wine) which is hiding the essence is only a form but the content is the essence.

17

The power of symbols is that the essence hidden in them is experienced unconsciously as immediately present and actual. If this does not happen, then it is not a symbol

A sign gives an indication. A stop sign, for instance, tells me what I should do. But stopping itself is not in the sign post. The sign has no power over me. Even a name plate is not a symbol, because it points to something different from itself, namely the person with that name but he is completely different from the name plate and might not even be present.

A symbol on the other hand represents the actual presence of the symbolised thing. In a symbol we are confronted directly but unconsciously with the hidden thing and the essence. For the conscious mind, the symbol is obscure and "unreal" because the meaning is hidden in the "other". For the unconscious it is entirely different: the "other" is precisely the expression of a whole which can never be reached by a definition of the conscious mind. The unconscious experiences and feels this whole through the symbol and does not think it as the conscious mind would.

Examples:

A dog symbolises male energy, a cat symbolises female energy. These conscious words say nothing to imply the diversity and emotional energy of a dog in its entirety. An encounter with a dog, whether in waking life or in a dream, is so complex and comprehensive that no analysis can hope to encompass all the chords that are touched.

Those aspects of the female energy that are symbolised by cats can never be described rationally. Any definition is a crass simplification. We have to actually touch a cat, feel its energy in order to sense the symbolic energy of its femininity.

It is quite a different thing to be with a living dog or cat as opposed to developing intelligent ideas about them. And it is precisely this direct encounter between living dynamic and energy-laden beings that takes place through symbols.

Symbols are irreplaceable, important and unique. The human conscious will never be able to replace symbols. As humans we can only conduct ourselves in our entirety thanks to symbols. We need symbols to reach our own reality and they give us intensity and wholeness. The interpretation of symbols helps us to perceive and understand the realities within ourselves better, but interpretation will never replace or rationalise symbols.

I distinguish between two types of symbols: **collective and individual.**

 Collective symbols are generally linked with human life and belong to the basic content of everyone's unconscious. These are for instance animal symbols such as cat and dog, cosmic symbols such as the sun and moon, the sphere, the tree of life, fruit, numbers and - **the body!**

An individual symbol can be anything that an individual wants it to be. The creation of an individual symbol is normally based on the specific experiences of that person which then get attached to a particular object. This object becomes the symbol and every time the person has contact with the object, he encounters or repeats his earlier experience. In other words, he re-enters the emotional energy zone connected with it.

What is typical of all symbols is that they directly affect the unconscious, completely independently of the conscious mind.

Allergy as an example of the functioning of symbols

The easiest way for me to explain how symbols work directly, immediately but entirely unconsciously, is by giving the example of allergies.

An allergy is the result of a repression of a spiritual problem that has been projected onto an external symbol.

In doing this, the unconscious normally uses collective symbols. These are identical symbols to those that occur in dreams. If a person dreams incessantly of dogs attacking him or if he develops a dog allergy, the issue is the same. The dog is the symbol of his problem.

If we repress an emotional problem, the unconscious identifies a symbol in the outside world that corresponds exactly to the problem. We give ourselves an allergy which means that we now have to avoid this symbol in the outside world too – the repression has now shifted to the exterior. By taking avoiding action we can suppress the symbol from our everyday life. However, this avoidance needs care and attention so that we are dealing all the time, albeit unconsciously, with our problem without of course solving it. In fact all this care is directed to repression and not to the solution of our problem.
Traditional medicine does not see or does not wish to see this cause and effect and deals with allergies by desensitising the patient. But the cause of the allergy is neither discovered nor solved by destroying a person's sensitivity.

An allergy appears when a spiritual problem arises and it disappears when that problem is solved.

Allergies show in a very impressive way how symbols function. The unconscious creates by spiritual means very strong physical defence mechanisms against things that are absolutely not injurious to the human organism. The fur of a cat or dog is not in any way aggressive. Dogs have been man's best friend and companion for

20

thousands of years. Apples, oranges and nuts are meant to be very healthy and positive for our well-being, but the unconscious is able to change the body so radically that very grave attacks occur when apples, oranges or nuts become symbols of repressed psychological problems. This connection is fascinating!

Everyone is able to recognise and solve the causes of his own allergy. This needs total honesty with oneself and the willingness to confront the problems that have been repressed into the unconscious. This honesty combined with some basic knowledge about the most important symbols enables everyone to sort himself out and to cure himself.

The following list – which is in no way complete – highlights some of the most frequent allergies, their symbolic meaning and the probable repressed problem.

Allergy to dogs:
In its widest sense a dog symbolises male energy or male persons (father, husband, brother...).   A dog allergy always indicates a conflict or emotional problem with male energy.

Women become allergic to dogs mostly as a reaction to a problem with their male partner. In men the allergy indicates a problem with their own masculinity.

The trigger for a dog allergy is always an actual man with whom the subject has had a specific experience. The archetypal man in our life is our father, both for men and women. That is why in the last instance a dog allergy always goes back to a problematic relationship with our father.

Allergy to cats:
A cat symbolises female energy from the aspect of female power and influence. In fairy tales a cat is often a witch's companion and "witchcraft" is symbolically present in cats: they are unpredictable, headstrong but soft and flattering and at the same time self-reliant and mystical.

A cat allergy is always an unconscious reaction to this kind of female energy. It generally refers to a fundamental problem with one's own mother. Women become allergic to cats if they deny or repress an important part of their femininity or fail to live it. For men it is because of a fear of female supremacy or in the end a fear of their mother. However, a cat allergy in men appears most frequently as a reaction to an actual female partner.

Allergy to horses
Fundamentally, the horse symbolises the sexual urge. I call the horse the "integrated urge". Young girls in puberty turn to horse riding when their sexuality awakens. Riding is an unconscious first approach to the actual sexual act and diffuses the girl's sexual energy through the horse... (There is a German saying that it is better to have a horse between one's legs than a man!!)
An allergy to horses is the expression of an unconscious problem with one's own sexual urge. If the urge cannot be fulfilled satisfactorily it is suppressed.

Allergy to nuts
Nuts symbolise the testicles and represent male sexual energy. A nut allergy is a reaction to an unconscious problem with male sexuality. In women, a nut allergy is often, but not always, a reaction to sexual abuse or to some other negative experience of male sexuality in childhood. The allergy might only erupt during a later relationship and can have its cause there (for example sexual rejection between partners).
If a man has a nut allergy the cause is a problem with his own sexuality (for instance impotence, fears, and inhibitions).

Hay fever
Hay fever is the expression of a deep-seated and repressed sadness. That is why the symptoms are identical to crying: weepy itchy eyes, a runny or blocked nose, irritated mucous membrane...
Hay fever is a reaction to pollen. The symbolism is easily understood: As long as the trees are bare during the dark season and the environment seems grey, sad and depressing, the environment is in harmony with the internal emotional mood of the subject. The blossoming of nature heralds a new beginning and a positive approach to life. This is exactly what the allergic person rejects. The

image of awakening life in nature contradicts his own sad frame of mind so that his unconscious makes his body react by "crying". He rejects the new bloom and exuberance because it is contrary to his own sorrowful state and makes it even more obvious to him.

Of course hay fever, like all allergies, has a trigger. Something happens that causes this repressed sorrow and unhappiness. This might be because of partners or children leaving, separations, house moving, other negative changes, unhappy partnerships or depressing professional situations. Find out for yourself!

Allergies to fruit and vegetables

Most fruit (cherries, strawberries, apples, oranges...) and many types of vegetables (cucumber, carrots and other penis shaped vegetables) are sexual symbols. The underlying cause of such an allergy is an unconscious sexual problem.

Milk allergy

Milk is associated unconsciously with our mother and motherhood. A milk allergy indicates an unconscious problem with our mother or with a person's own maternal instinct.

Other foodstuffs

Allergies to food are nowadays so widespread and some of them are so specific, that I cannot deal with them all. As a rule, I would recommend that one should take a serious look at the relationship to the mother, in particular in cases involving children. It is essentially the mother's role to feed the child – and most especially to feed the child emotionally – so that it seems to me that the cause of many food allergies is an unconscious emotional problem with one's mother. In adults it can be helpful to ask who the food provider is and whether there is an unconscious problem there.

Allergy to house dust

This form of allergy is a reaction to a feeling of being rejected by one or both parents. A house dust allergy is caused by the belief that "I am not good enough"; "I do not measure up to my parents' expectations"; "I do everything wrong, I *am* wrong, that is why I am always being criticised".

23

House dust is natural. If everything has to be clinically clean and by inference harsh rules and expectations are laid down within the family, even unconsciously, the child will feel that these have to be adhered to as a precondition of his parents' love. House dust becomes a symbol: Something is wrong with me! This is not allowed! This is dusty or dirty, I am not "clean" enough...

An allergy to house dust is basically an expression of an emotional problem with one or both parents and is always combined with an inferiority complex.

Allergies to metals

In my experience, this type of allergy is connected with a negative experience with a very specific person. This person would have been wearing metal as a chain, ring, button, cuff link, key or something similar.

Frightening experiences involving metals, or metal instruments, as for instance operations, can also be the cause of such allergies. It is mostly very difficult to reconstruct an event that has been deeply suppressed into the unconscious (for example sexual abuse or other negative childhood experiences such as beatings or humiliation). The unconscious links this repressed experience with that specific metal and reacts allergically. An allergy to metal is an attempt to sublimate a bad experience connected unconsciously with that metal but generally identified with a person.

The body – a complete symbolic system

The body is a complete system of symbols for the unconscious, which means that every part of the body and every organ has a designated symbolic meaning. Just as dogs, cats, horses, nuts etc. that exist outside of us, have definite symbolic meanings, all the parts of our body also have specific symbolic significance.

There are many sayings which have developed over the years that refer to parts of the body and their symbolism.
The nose indicates knowledge (or the lack of it) and hence self-perception, viz. "As plain as the nose on your face" "Under one's very nose" "Poke one's nose into everything".
The gall and the bile are associated with bitterest grief.
An old superstition held that the blood in the liver of a sacrificed animal before a battle had to be blood-red to be favourable, but if it was pale, it augured defeat. Hence a coward was called "white-livered or lily-livered".
"To bring someone to their knees" expresses defeat, humiliation and subordination.
"Shit-scared" graphically describes the body's reaction to fear.
"Having words stuck in one's throat" means being unable to utter the words that then are repressed.

In general, very few people are aware of these connotations passed on to us through old sayings.

The significance of some parts of the body & disease.

The human body can be regarded as being in two halves, the right and the left.
In principle, **the left side** represents our emotional and feminine side. An illness in the left upper part of the body generally indicates an emotional problem connected with our relationships, including our relationship to our self. (Example: heart attack)

The **right side** of the body represents our rational and masculine side and our relationship with the wider world.
An illness in the right side of the body indicates that a consciously taken decision is posing a problem for us. Likewise, the right side stands for our work and all our activities in the wider world.

The human body can be seen as a time-and-development scale divided into sections of seven years, going from set to set of large joints and beginning at the feet. The foot itself, however, from the sole to the ankle, is an exception and represents the first year of life, or in other words the time we need to adapt to our arrival in the world. Thus, the body corresponds from the feet to the head, to a natural order of the general tasks of mankind.

The **first year of our life** takes place against the background of our arrival on earth. Our task in this new life is to gain confidence ("to get our feet on the ground") and to hit it off with our parents. The left foot up to the ankle represents our first year's relationship to our mother and the right foot that to our father.

The **first seven years of our life**, symbolised by the section from sole to knee, represent our actual childhood. The most impressive experiences are made during this period with our parents (left leg with mother, right leg with father.) We learn how to interact with the family and society (socialisation) and we develop our set of beliefs about our self, life and the wider world. Around the 7th year, we are sent to school and our early childhood in its narrowest sense is thus actually over. We leave the close circle of the family and, for the first time, we have to enter and adapt to a wider society represented through school. Our childish ego is thus "bent", which is represented symbolically by the knees.

The years from 7 to 14 are symbolised by the section from knee to hip joint. We go to school and become part of a larger society. Puberty intervenes around 14, the genital region alters, pubic hair grows and we are transformed into young adults (the trunk of our body). Up till now we defined ourselves in relation to our mother (left leg) and our father (right leg). This now stops. We now need to become our own person and develop our own personality. Symbolically, the hip joint kicks in and, being the largest joint in our body, it represents the largest enduring change in our life.

The **years from 14 to 21** represent our puberty – in our simile this would be the core of the body, from the sexual organs to the neck. We need to rebel against our parents and their values, their standards, ideas and behaviour in order to find ourselves. We fight everything that is old or traditional, we test our limits and often overstep the mark in order to prove ourselves. The bladder and the intestines symbolise this action of letting old values go. This is the cue: letting go of parental ties! Our aggressions manifest themselves strongly (liver, gall, acne) and first love smites us in this period (heart). Most of all, we need to redefine our internal attitude to life. After all these conflicts, we must accept ourselves in our newly defined life (lungs). Once we have succeeded in this process, we have become adults.

The **years from 21 to 28** are shaped by nature to make us create solid and lasting relationships, to produce children (left upper arm) and to find our place in the professional world – education, studies – (right upper arm).

In **the years from 28 to 36** we consolidate our position in a partnership or our own family and in our job. As a partner or father and mother (left lower arm) or as a working person (right lower arm) we have stabilised our existence. The hands symbolise the idea that it is only in this phase of our life that we really can give and take. Before, we were only learning about relationships and work. Now, however, we have sorted out a balance between giving and receiving.

The **years from 35 to 42**, symbolised by the throat or neck, challenge us to recognise and formulate our own desires. Until this phase in our life, we tended to follow the values and standards of others, mainly of our parents, without questioning them very much. We now begin to wonder what we really want and whether what we have done so far is fulfilling us. "What do I really want?" is the question that characterises this phase. Slowly, we learn to recognise our own needs and to define them against the background of our situation. Some wide ranging corrections may have to be undertaken, because until now we have oriented ourselves too much according to the expectations of other people. Partnerships and the choice of jobs are now scrutinised. Parenthood becomes a challenge as the children grow up and throw up new problems.

The **years between 42 and 49** are the hardest because life gives us the difficult task of *knowing ourselves*. In the simile of the body, this phase is represented by the face from the chin to the crown of the head. It is only this late in life that we look seriously at ourselves. Everything is still just at our disposal. This can be the so-called "mid-life crisis". We ask ourselves: "What am I really doing here?" when we examine our work-a-day life and our relationships. Problems that we have so far hidden away in the background now surface and haunt us. Honest self-knowledge is now of paramount importance without which we fall ill. This is the time for the last big changes. Maybe a new profession? If yes, then this is the time to jump because a new start becomes more difficult or even impossible as time goes on. Separation? Should I really break up the partnership or the family? Conflicts become more obvious and cannot be brushed away anymore. The consequences of our earlier decisions are clearer and cannot be suppressed, although it is hard to look at them (our eyesight begins to fail). This is the time of the first true harvest of our life. We are compelled to see what has happened to our efforts; who we are and where we honestly stand. We have to recognise that everything that we did and decided has had a lasting effect on us and is irreversible. The real seriousness of our life hits us powerfully because we realise that we are experiencing the consequences of all our previous decisions.

From our 49th year on, we reach maturity which should transform itself into wisdom. Looking back we also aspire to a higher kind of future associated with spirituality. Our body has reached and passed the apex of its development and it now slowly but inexorably retrenches. Growing older gives us the opportunity also to become calmer and more balanced. We needn't prove anything to anyone anymore. This is the time of maturity. Spiritual questions and insights shape this phase. The crown of the head (the fontanelle) is the opening in our body pointing "upwards" or to the spiritual world of the "hereafter", where we all go after death and from where we all came. We prepare ourselves to close that circle and to take as much wisdom and maturity along as we possibly can. The material world slowly loses its interest for us while we devote ourselves more to intellectual and spiritual aspects.

Symbolic meaning of some organs and illnesses

In the following I have made an alphabetical list of some parts of the body, organs and illnesses in order to illustrate their symbolic meaning.

Accidents

Although it is difficult for many people to comprehend, we actually create our own accidents (see also up "The power of creation"). Accidents are rooted in an excess of aggression directed against ourselves. The trigger for an accident is a belief in violence in the unconscious, either violence against our self or against someone who has annoyed us intensely. Whatever the reason, an accident is always self-punishment. We do violence to ourselves with the help of other things or seemingly innocent bystanders. The part of the body injured gives us a clue as to the interpretation of the accident. What can the person not do anymore? In what way has he been incapacitated? Or what has he managed to gain from the injury (for example rest)?

People who often have accidents (fractures, wounds, sprains etc.) are storing up too many aggressions. They belong to a group of people who have a very harsh and critical value system (directed also at themselves). But most of all, they tend to run down their own feelings and in particular their aggressions. In order to reduce their likelihood of having accidents it is necessary for them to look closely and honestly at their own feelings and particularly at their rage!

Let your rage in! Find out what makes you cross! Allow yourself to feel negative feelings and to think negative thoughts – that is how they can flow away. If they are bottled up, these feelings erupt in an accident and turn against you.

Questions:

What organ or part of the body is affected? Hence:
What current problem is at the bottom of this?
Who is making me feel so very angry at the moment?
Why am I punishing myself instead of others?

Acne

Acne gives a simple message: "I don't want to grow up!" – "I am frightened of becoming an adult!" – "I cannot cope with taking full responsibility for my own life!" Acne is associated with puberty, which is when we distance ourselves from our parents' rules, fight them and train ourselves to resist so that we can find ourselves and grow up. So every little pimple is a small aggression, a sort of outburst of rage experienced on the skin and thus not consciously given an outlet in development and growth. The unconscious background for acne is a conflict with one or both parents, an unresolved opposition or resistance to mother or father. The opposition may be directed at substitute figures (boss, partner) but it is always retraceable to an unresolved relationship to a parent in teen-age years. No matter how old the person is, it means that he or she is emotionally stuck in puberty.

Questions:

> *Why do I not want to grow up?*
> *Which one of my parents am I actually opposed to?*
> *What constraints stop me from cutting loose?*
> *What do I see as the negative aspects of being in charge of my own destiny?*
> *What sacrifices have I made internally?*
> *Is it really easier to continue to internally defy my parents?*

Alcoholism

This is a flight from a sad and depressing situation in life. An alcoholic tries to anaesthetize himself. He imagines that he cannot be happy, relaxed and content without numbing himself. A deep-seated emotional problem, a feeling of sorrow and resignation depress him utterly. Alcoholism is a very simple way to drown one's sorrows.

Questions:

> *What is the true reason for my emotional problem?*
> *What makes me so sad and disappointed?*
> *What bothers me in my situation in life?*
> *Why do I think I need to numb myself?*
> *What am I trying to run away from: conflict, change?*

31

Angina

Angina is a reaction to frustrations and aggressions that have not been expressed. Someone has pained us or irritated us. This injury burns like a fire in our throat. But it is not only the injury that burns, but also the resulting aggressions burn us because they cannot be off-loaded.

Hurtful words are held back but they now stick in our throat (see "throat").

Questions:

> *Who do I feel has hurt me just now?*
> *What has hit me so hard emotionally that I feel it is stuck in my throat?*
> *What insult is just too much for me to swallow?*
> *What aggressive words welled up inside me, but I forced them back?*

Arms

The left arm represents grasping, giving and taking in our relationships, and in particular in our partnerships. If we have unconscious problems with our partner, children, mother or other close associate, the left arm may suffer.

The right arm represents gripping, taking and giving in our work environment and the "world" of our conscious decisions. If we have problems at work, with seizing opportunities, with providing solutions or with making decisions, the right arm may suffer.

Arthritis

This disease indicates that a person's internal approach to life has become stuck in a rut. We have become set on a particular view. This stiff attitude manifests itself in our joints. It is interesting to note in what joints the arthritis first appears. Our joints symbolise our mental ability to change direction in life. If our joints become stiff and inflexible, it means that they are reacting to a certain mental or spiritual inflexibility which was always present, and that this lies at the cause of the complaint. If the intellect or spirit becomes stiff, rigid and inflexible, the body will follow suit. It means that there is an internal resistance to positive changes, there is a lack of vision and no wish for change.

Questions:

> *Why do I want to hold on to an unsatisfactory situation?*
> *Why am I so frightened of change?*
> *Why am I directing my defiance against myself?*
> *What do I really want?*
> *What is my positive vision for a good life?*
> *What stops me from believing that change is possible?*

Asthma

Asthma is a bodily reaction to excessive emotional pressure exerted by a close person. In childhood it is almost always one or both parents who exert this emotional pressure that the child cannot fend off. That is why asthma often abates when the afflicted person leaves home. The sufferer feels in the truest sense of the word that his "breath is taken away". This emotional pressure can have various causes such as high levels of performance expected by the parents or perhaps a certain neediness of one or other parent: "You must help me emotionally".

Questions:

> *What person in my close circle takes my breath away?*
> *What kind of pressure really bothers me emotionally?*
> *Who has too much power over me? (father, mother, partner).*

Back

Our back or our spinal column, being our body's main support, symbolises the unconscious feeling of being well or badly adjusted and supported in our life. Our back suffers if we unconsciously believe that we are in a situation where we do not have enough support from others or from life. It also suffers if we feel that too much is "heaped on" us or that we have overburdened ourselves. In this case, it is an orthopaedic problem, in other words, the support system is reacting pathologically.

Our back also symbolises old things, things that are behind us. If we have problems with old hurts that we no longer wish to see, these can appear as tumours or skin and nerve complaints on the back.

If the shoulder muscles are tensed up, the sufferer is probably under a lot of pressure. Tenseness is always a reaction to pressure and stress. We cannot "loosen up". Left shoulder tense: pressure and stress in a relationship; right shoulder: pressure and stress at work or over a conscious decision.

Bladder
The bladder is symbolically associated with letting go, just as it is physically. It becomes diseased if we cannot let an emotional injury go. The causes are normally in our close circle: father/mother/partner/children. The bladder is like a store room for our feelings of victimisation. We retain in our bladder insults, perceived offences, hurtful situations where we have felt unloved, used, abandoned or attacked. Bladder infections in women are often connected with their relationship with their father - and a male partner might re-ignite this relationship.
Questions:
> *When exactly did this bladder problem start?*
> *What hurtful event took place with father or partner?*
> *What old hurtful situations with father/mother come to mind in this connection?*
> *Do I really want to nurse this grudge and continue to feel like a victim?*

Blood pressure
   • **High blood pressure**
Aggression and feelings of permanent pressure and disadvantage want to surface but are not allowed to. The person is "pressurised". These feelings are suppressed, and pressure produces counter-pressure, which is exactly what high blood pressure is all about. This is a complaint that mainly affects people with a very strict and narrow value system, people who judge themselves and others

severely. They tend to discount their own feelings. For them, feelings are a sign of weakness, which is why they do not admit to themselves that at times they feel aggressive, disadvantaged, pressured or humiliated. Inside them there is a boiling cauldron of unconscious rage. A person with high blood pressure constantly forces himself to increase his performance in order to gain recognition, but this finally plays on his nerves and makes him aggressive as a means of compensation.

- **Low blood pressure**

A person with low blood pressure is afraid of his own vital impulses. I call the aggressive feelings and other impulses within the unconscious that the sufferer deems dangerous "vital impulses". This fear of one's own aggressions or of all the vital, animalistic and wild urges in one's personality is backed by yet another deeper fear, namely a fear of getting involved in conflicts and the resulting separations that might occur. Low blood pressure is the body's way of saying that vital impulses, especially aggressions that are needed for dealing normally with life, are being repressed. In a way, low blood pressure can be regarded as resignation, like saying: "There is no point in making an effort", or "I have given up trying to make something of my life..."

Brain

The brain represents our "controller", our rudder and our governing body. It is our alert and vigilant consciousness and enables us to make adult value judgments. Brain disorders generally indicate an acute desire to step away mentally from one's situation in life.

- **Meningitis.**

Meningitis is based on an inflammatory family situation that the sufferer wishes to escape from. The message is: "I cannot continue to live with the conflict that the constellation of my family has put me in!" Meningitis is an attempt to flee. The sufferer is the carrier of symptoms of a larger conflict within the family and he or she is no longer able to withstand the pressure. He shuts his mind, so to speak, and the necessary stay in hospital takes him away from his family, providing a salutary side-effect.

Questions:

> *What family conflict is the cause of the illness?*
> *What particular part do I play within it?*
> *What expectation of/by parents or other relatives are behind that?*
> *Whose suffering /pain/ problem do I think I need to bear?*

- **Brain aneurism**

Bleeding in the brain that leads to long-term damage and disability is an expression of the unconscious refusal to grow up and to take full responsibility for one's life. As a rule, the sufferer returns to a childlike state. The disability returns the person to his family or to an environment resembling his family. A deep desire to regress lies at the bottom of such serious haemorrhages of the brain. The person wishes to get out of adulthood and does this by excessive bleeding.

Questions:

> *Why do I want to get out and refuse to be an adult?*
> *What makes it so difficult for me to accept full responsibility for my life?*
> *How have I come to feel a failure as an adult?*

- **Brain tumour**

A brain tumour is a self-punishment for failing to reach a level of achievement that one has set far too high for oneself. Very controlled people who attribute much too much weight to their reason tend to punish themselves. The "controller" turns against his own health. In terms of the conscious mind, a brain tumour corresponds to suicide by a shot to the head.

Questions:

> *What exactly are my unconscious demands on myself?*
> *For what particular failure am I condemning myself at present?*
> *How can I soften my very firm set of values and make positive changes?*
> *What set of beliefs about myself is behind this affliction?*
> *What do I need to forgive myself for?*

Breast

A woman's breast may be affected if she feels unconsciously that she is made to give too much and gets very little in return .The function of the breast is to provide for another life. It is essential to the new-born baby. It keeps another being alive.

The breast has of course also an erotic function but in my experience this aspect is of minor importance in breast cancer, for example. Emotionally, a breast disorder, particularly cancer, is triggered by a feeling of being used or of being the victim. *"I am always there for others, but no-one bothers about me!" "I keep on giving, but nothing comes back to me. On the contrary, I feel more and more used up emotionally..."; "I sacrifice myself for others (children, partner, colleagues, parents...) but I am taken for granted..."* – These are the beliefs and feelings that lie at the core of breast disorders (that can also affect men).

- **Breast cancer**:

The aggression resulting from frustration directs itself against the woman. Cancer is an aggression that should be directed at others but is not materialised and therefore attacks itself.

Questions:

When exactly did this disorder affect the body? What was happening before that? (1, 2, or more years before)?
Which breast is affected –right or left?
Left breast: I will look honestly at my relationship with my children and my mother – When do I feel like a victim? Am I taken for granted? Do I keep giving and never get anything back?
Right breast: I will look honestly at my relationship with my husband (or with men), with my colleagues and my father – When do I feel like a victim? Am I taken for granted? Do I keep giving and never get anything back?
My feelings of victimisation are honest and I recognise my aggression against those people to whom I have given too much and who do not reciprocate at all or insufficiently.

I will look honestly at the unconscious model I follow that leads me always to help and be there for others. I will dig deeper and examine my inferiority complex and try to discover why I always find myself in a situation where there is imbalance between giving and taking.

Cancer

Cancer signifies that the body is suffering as a result of a person's awakening death wish based on aggression. This aggressive and destructive behaviour is clearly identifiable physically because the patient's own cells transform themselves and begin to attack and eat up their host. This dynamic shows very clearly that the main emotion which has the strongest influence is repressed aggression. Such a potent and devastating self-aggression can have many causes. Very often it is a deep sense of guilt. In this case the aggression contained in the cancer is self-punishment. The sufferer accuses him or herself for some failure or inadequacy (for example cancer of the womb, brain tumour, prostate cancer). Other causes may be disappointment or deep sorrow. Our psychological energy rules that every frustration creates aggression. Sadness is always coupled with disillusionment in our unconscious. In this way sad experiences are transformed into aggressions. If disillusion and sadness lie at the bottom of our aggression, the cancer will attack certain organs like the bowel, stomach, pancreas or the breast.

A further cause may be a fundamental resignation; the person is fed up with his life, it has no more meaning for him - in which case he would probably direct the cancer to his lungs.

Cancer is based on one or several experiences that have raised such negative emotions that one's own life seems in some way no longer worth living. The aggression, conditioned by frustration, cannot surface to the conscious level because of anxiety and negative thought patterns, nor can it erupt and thus be diffused, so that it starts to gnaw at the person himself.

When a cancerous growth is discovered, it is very important to know where the primary infection started, because this will indicate what the underlying repression is. Time is also a factor. The cancer patient should try to look back at least over the last two years before falling ill, and sometimes it is useful to look back even further: what happened then?

It is important to bring the repressed feelings – in particular aggressions – into the conscious mind in order to restore good health.

Questions:

> *Which organ is affected? (see IV. The significance of some parts of the body and disease)*
> *Exactly when was the illness first noted?*
> *What happened before the illness broke out?*
> *What changes or misfortunes took place?*
> *What repressed feelings might be the cause of the cancer?*
> *What can I do to experience and live through these feelings consciously?*
> *What do I need to make my life worth living again?*
> *Am I prepared to opt unreservedly to live life?*
> *Am I prepared to stop feeling that I am a victim?*

Children's illnesses

People ask me very often whether all these symbolic meanings of disease also apply to children, seeing that they are still so small! It is exactly because they are so small that they need to use their body to express their problems. The less developed the conscious mind, the more the body becomes the instrument to express problems.

The human consciousness takes about 12 years to grow to maturity. The younger the child, the more important it is in my view to apply the knowledge I have described here to discover the underlying problems, in particular if the child is still too small to speak or think clearly.

It seems to me that the "normal" children's illnesses (mumps, chicken pox, German measles, measles...) are a kind of body rehearsal for the challenges of life. These diseases make the child develop antibodies that make him stronger and increase his defences. Of course these illnesses all carry a risk – just as life does. Children are now vaccinated against most of these. Personally, I feel that we are taking away children's ability to become strong and to develop their own antibodies. In short, we are making our children weak. I would tend to let children have these childhood diseases so that they

39

confront life challenges in this way and become strong and able to stay healthy later on.

Conjunctivitis

The conjunctiva becomes inflamed if we see something at the moment that irritates and annoys us. The energy of the inflammation corresponds with our rage. The eye is saying symbolically: *"I am annoyed by what I see!"* Left eye: what is currently happening in my partnership or in my close relationships? Right eye: What is currently happening in my work? Which conscious decisions have I made that annoy me?

Coughing

I shall bark at the world to rid myself of my aggressions! Something does not suit me but I cannot find words to say so. Coughing is a way of ejecting a current unhappy feeling (see respiratory organs) A person draws attention to himself by coughing: *"Are you listening? I am barking at you! I am truly fed up with something but I cannot tell you what because it makes me scared."*
Questions:

> *What exactly is making you so discontent at the moment?*
> *Who am I actually barking at? Who is making me feel aggressive?*
> *In what situations does my cough attack me?*
> *When does my cough quieten down?*
> *Who do I irritate by coughing?*

Death

Some illnesses frequently end in death, for example cancer. Death is our ultimate means of escaping from a conflict or an unresolved problem. This is why we have within us a death wish. We can decide to die. Many of the so-called fatal illnesses are a result of us unconsciously activating our death wish.
Death through illness is based on an unconscious decision to die. This decision is not always clear-cut so that the death wish and the

40

survival instinct fight each other and a long period of suffering ensues. The clearer the unconscious decision to die is, the faster we succumb. The clearer the unconscious decision to live is, the faster we get better. I do not believe in fatal diseases. I believe that we can turn around every disease into life and health. For this, a clear and strong decision in the unconscious must be made. For it is in the unconscious that the power lies to opt for life or death. Many people repress their true emotional conflicts and problems for years until they finally resign themselves unconsciously to never finding any answers. This is the moment when for instance cancer takes hold. Instead of positively changing a depressing life situation, people opt for resignation and hence disease or even death.

Diabetes

The message of diabetes is: My life has lost its sweetness. The illness can be understood as a depression suppressed into the **pancreas**. Something has happened to make me sad and it has taken hold of my entire life force. That is why diabetes often also affects the eyes: I refuse to see what happened and made me so sad, Diabetes is a depressive resignation that has been transferred to the body. "My life is no longer sweet and lovely – that's the way it is... I am resigned to it...there is nothing I can do...

Questions:

> *What happened to make my life so sad?*
> *What do I need to make my life sweet again?*
> *What changes must I make to enjoy life again?*
> *Why am I resigned and why don't I believe in change any more?*
> *Is it too much effort to change my life myself?*
> *Do I wish to spend the rest of my life in this resignation or am I brave enough to make positive changes?*

Disabilities (inborn)

Inborn disabilities affecting either the body or the mind are, according to the state of my knowledge, the result of an earlier life and conditioned by karma. It is a very restrictive fallacy to believe

41

that we only live once. We have several hundred lives and the central thread of our identity winds through all our previous incarnations. We do not appear in this world as a blank page but bring along manifold experiences and unresolved problems too.

An inborn disability is not necessarily the outcome of an earlier life, but can also be produced by the embryo. A baby might well refuse sight in his new incarnation and therefore be born blind. We make decisions in every phase of our existence – before life, in life and after life. We can therefore make decisions at any time and in any reality and these might – even with a time lapse – take the shape of disease or disability at a material level.

Every life makes specific demands on our learning. A person who is born disabled has to develop a special learning process in this existence which we need to respect. These connections which I call karma are often associated in our western civilisation with "blame" or "punishment" for evil deeds in an earlier life. I would plead that such moral judgements are entirely misplaced. A disabled person has been assigned a very special task in this life, we do not know why, but the reason can only be ascertained within the person himself.

Ears

Our ears of course are symbolically our hearing. They become unwell if we do not wish to hear something.

- **Otitis** and similar infections:

I refuse to hear what is being said to me: words of criticism, antagonism, separation, demands etc. Children suffer from ear infections if they are often criticised or their parents argue a lot or other words are spoken (or even only thought) by other people that they would rather not hear.

Questions:
> *What words from outside do I not wish to hear at present?*
> *Was I being criticised? If so, by whom?*
> *Do other people say nasty things about me? (maybe not within my hearing)*
> *What do I simply not want to hear currently?*

- **Tinnitus** (a constant ringing in the ears):

I do not want to hear my own voice. Tinnitus is always the result of suppressing one's own inner warning voice. This voice only raises itself if we treat ourselves badly, overtax ourselves or burn ourselves out by taking a negative path. In order to drown out this voice, the sufferer creates a din or a tinnitus in his ears. In this way the body cancels out the inner warning voice. In extremely severe cases, hearing loss occurs which is a consequence of the situation I have just described: I do not want to hear my own voice, I will cancel it out.

Questions:

> *Why am I so stubborn that I refuse to listen to my own inner voice?*
> *Why do I cling to this path which is wrong? (Ambition? Professional aspiration? Need for security...?)*
> *Why am I so frightened of change?*

- **Behind the ears**

This is where our earliest childhood feelings are located *("You are still wet behind the ears!")* If we have problems behind the ears (for example eczema, rash, lichen and similar skin diseases), it means that we are in a situation where we are recalling feelings from our infancy that we have not worked through. Problems behind the left ear normally indicate emotions relating to our mother, whereas the right ear relates to our father.

Questions:

> *What feelings from my early childhood wish to be heard?*
> *Who in my close environment has activated these feelings?*
> *What exactly do I still need to work through emotionally regarding my mother or father?*

43

Eating disorders
- **Over- eating.**

Emotional neediness is the psychological cause of over-eating. "I am not getting enough love and affection" is what the subject feels. At the same time, corpulence provides protection against further injury or attack. Eating is a displacement therapy. What cannot be gained emotionally or psychologically, such as love, understanding, affection and safety, is acquired orally with the intake of food. If a person finds that the people around him are cold, aggressive or domineering, he eats, and his padding will also protect him from further attacks and from the "cold world".

As a rule, two types of character tend to eat as a substitute:

Relationship-oriented people have a basic problem, in that they are not naturally aggressive, they cannot impose their will nor can they say "No!" They let themselves be used, they are the helpers, the do-gooders, but in the long run they sense an imbalance between their loving sacrifice for the advantage of others and their own needs. Not enough love, affection and recognition seem to flow back to them. This frustration is off-set by eating. Over-eating is an addiction like alcoholism. People believe that by eating, they are rewarding themselves for their goodness and they comfort themselves with food. The short-term sensuous pleasure replaces their frustration. Their mindset is: "I am not worthy of love, others are worthier than I am; I never get any love, I am unloved..."

The second group are order or power-oriented people. The basic problem is identical: insufficient love, affection, warmth and acknowledgement. They use food to overcome their frustration by giving themselves internal and external protection or padding. They grumble, they are never satisfied, they are domineering and seem impossible to please. Eating is again replacement therapy, but with a strong aggressive note: The mindset is: *"I am bad and unloved; the world is rotten and unfair; I never get a chance; I always have to fight for my rights; I am not lovable..."*

Diets never work because a positive change is required in the negative set of beliefs that lie at the bottom of this eating disorder.

- **Not eating enough (Anorexia)**

This indicates resignation about life: "I *don't want to be here; it is pointless to make any effort; I   am not entitled to live.*" Anorexia is a massive lack of self-worth. Eating too little is an escape or a resigned defeat. A feeling of being fundamentally overburdened by life and not being able to cope is also possibly a psychological cause of this eating disorder.

Elbow

Our elbows represent change of direction. They suffer if we resist changing the direction of our thoughts and actions in a concrete situation. The left elbow reacts to a resistance in the relationship sphere, especially in partnerships. The right elbow reacts to a resistance in the work sphere and our conscious decisions.
Questions:

> *What change in direction in my life am I currently resisting?*
> *What change is being imposed on me from outside that I do not want?*

Epilepsy

This illness belongs to a small group of disorders that are caused by spiritual possession (see also spleen and schizophrenia). A spirit from outside has penetrated the subject and now lives within him or her. The subject is responsible himself, in that he has opened himself up to this penetration. Some event has caused an opening, making it possible for a destructive, foreign body to enter. The event may be alcohol, sexual excesses, spiritual experiments (such as Reiki-sessions or similar) post-partum vacuum in women and other illnesses or crises.

Traditional medicine is not able to cure epilepsy which is plausible once we know that the cause is spiritual. It follows therefore that epilepsy can only be cured spiritually, for example through prayer, ceremonies etc, and here the wholehearted participation of the afflicted person plays an important part

Eyes

The eyes become diseased if there is something we do not wish to see.

- **Short-sightedness** (myopia) occurs against a background of interior resistance to seeing

something that has happened and has a lasting problematic effect. Children become short-sighted when siblings are born, when they are sent to kindergarten, when their parents divorce, school starts, they move house etc.

Adults become short-sighted when they have come to the end of their studies and worry about their future (fearing it may not be what they want) or when they get married in spite of being internally unsure of the decision; or when they have children although they subconsciously regard them as a limitation and an encumbrance. So there is always a reality that intervenes but which we do not want to see and which is likely to endure unless we change it.

- **Far-sightedness**

This relates to a problem in the present: There is something in my life at present that I do not wish to see, so I shall look into the distance, i.e. into the future. I find it difficult to look at that which is close up, in my immediate present. Middle age or old age far-sightedness (presbyopia) starts generally after forty years of age. This is when we become more and more aware that our present situation is a consequence of our earlier decisions. The older we get, the more limited our sphere of action becomes, because the result of our choices (choice of job, partner, children, work place) stack up "behind" us like a hill. It becomes more difficult or almost impossible in old age to change an existing situation. If the present is not satisfactory or fulfilling, we turn our eyes into an imaginary "future" i.e. into the far distance.

- **Cross-eyed**

Being cross-eyed indicates a skewed attitude to reality and to life: I do not want to see things as they really are – and this mind set is very pronounced.

- **Blindness**

The realities or things that the afflicted person would like to be rid of have become so ingrained that he refuses to see them at all. Blindness is retreat and resignation. Instead of recognising that these realities are created by himself, the sufferer gives up trying actively to change them and chooses instead blindness: *"I can't look at them anymore! I refuse to see them! Once and for all!"*
Questions:
> *Exactly when did the eye troubles start?*
> *What happened before that time?*
> *What active steps can I take to change my situation?*
> *What decisions are required to change my life positively?*

Family illnesses

In some families, the same illnesses repeat themselves, such as cancer, depression, hair loss etc. Traditional medicine explains this with the genes. I explain it with the unconscious assimilation of the repressions of the parents by the children. All children tend to copy the unconscious fears and beliefs of their parents, both consciously and unconsciously. These fears constitute the basic emotional "energy field" of the child. Example: The parents went through the bombings and starvation of war. This gave them fears about their actual existence. The children pick up these fears without ever having faced a similar situation. Just like their parents, the children now develop a very strong need for safety, they find it difficult to let go or to throw things away, preferring to hoard things etc. This is how certain characteristics develop in a family and in the long run even in a nation.

Family illnesses run along the same lines. Parents unconsciously show their children by example how to deal with feelings. Because everything takes place at an unconscious level, the children are unconsciously informed and shaped by the knowledge of the disease of their elders. The way that feelings are repressed is generally passed on in families. That is why the result of these repressions is a recurrence of the same illnesses. In families that repress mainly aggressions, cancer tends to be the most general form of its pathological expression. In families that demand high performance

47

(even if this is not discussed openly but even more so if it is simply expected), the male members are quite likely to suffer hair loss, high blood pressure and probably die of heart attacks. Families that harbour feelings of victimisation will be prone to bladder disorders, depression and similar illnesses. Families that pass on emotional pressures, often experience recurrent cases of asthma etc.

Recurrent illnesses in a family show how that family deals with feelings and emotional problems.

Another reason for family illnesses is when a child substitutes himself for a parent. Many childrens' complaints are substitute illnesses within the framework of the family. This can be very serious and even lead to death if a parent wishes to leave the family. ("Before you go, mother/father, I want to go!") Some children basically fall ill and stay ill, in order to save the family from break-up. I can only point briefly to the complicated connections between family members in this context. I cannot deal with these intricacies here, but in my experience each case should be looked at very carefully.

Feet

Feet show our standing in life. If our feet fail, we cannot walk nor stand. We cannot move forward and we are blocked. If we cannot even stand, our whole standing in life is adversely affected

- **Athletes' foot**

Fungus only appears in nature on rotting or dead material. If we create a fungal infection, it refers to an old emotional problem. We can discover what it is about by its location on the foot (see toes). Athletes' foot indicates an old fundamental emotion, an old injury or a wound that is "eating away" at us.

- **Left foot:** relationships/ partnership/ mother
- **Right foot**: work/conscious decisions/father
- **Toe nails**: protection: Where do I feel unprotected? Where might my protection tear?
- **Sole of the foot**: problems with my standing in life; problems rooted in my past.

48

Questions:
> *Where do I not want to go at the moment?*
> *What is blocking me from moving forward?*
> *What is making it difficult for me to stand up for myself?*

Fingers
The thumb stands for our worries.
Index finger: stands for fear and our ego.
Middle finger: stands for aggression and sexuality (finger sign meaning "fuck you!")
Ring finger: stands for our bonds and separations.
Little finger: stands for the part we play in our family (both in our ancestral and present family).
As before, the left hand: relationships, mother; right hand: work/ world or relationship to father/male partner.
Finger nails: protection. Where do I feel unprotected? Where might my protection tear?

Fungus (see also athletes' foot in section on feet)
Fungus grows on dying or dead tissue in nature. If fungus appears on the body, it signals something old: an old injury that we wish to repel and that is also often repellent to others (because it is also contagious.) Fungus eats us and gnaws at us. The question is: what part of the body is affected? This can help to understand the underlying problem. If the vagina is affected, a resistance against the present sexual partner may be the cause. Fungus, as such, implies an older wound. In this instance, it is worthwhile looking beyond the present partner and to ask about the woman's own father and to investigate whether some injury (maybe a sexual one) occurred.

Gall

The gall bladder represents the processing of aggression. It falls ill if we repress our aggressions over a long period ("The gall of bitterness"). A disorder of the gall often means that we have a deep belief that stops us from being normally and naturally aggressive, a mindset that says: "I always have to be the goodie".
Questions:

> *Who has been annoying me so much?*
> *What enrages me so much although I cannot admit it?*

Haemorrhages

Blood is the sap of life and symbolises the free-flowing joy of life. If our blood is diseased we lose our joy of life. Haemorrhages mean that our body is weeping. Life itself is crying within us when we bleed. Every drop of blood is a tear-drop of life. This is deepest grief, deeper than tears.
Questions:

> *Which organ is bleeding? (See IV.The significance of some parts of the body and disease))*
> *What emotional wound is the cause of this bleeding?*
> *What makes me so very sad that I must weep blood?*

Haemorrhoids

This relates to an old injury in a relationship that one refuses to get over or rid oneself of (bowel movement). If there is bleeding, it means that we are crying when we have to let go. The underlying cause is a feeling of guilt and an attitude that says: "It is preferable to keep the pain than to have nothing at all."
Questions:

> *What wound do I wish to hang on to through pain?*
> *Why do I find it so difficult to let go?*

Hair

Hair represents strength and vigour. Hair loss is a physical reaction to spiritual stress and emotional pressure. The cause is feeling that is overburdened or overtaxed: "I just can't manage! Too much is expected of me!"...

In our performance driven culture, the pressures are becoming ever greater, and more and more young men are becoming bald or have thin hair. Women lose their hair in stressful or pressurised professions or if their life imposes such stresses. Marriage or childbirth can also exert emotional pressure and cause hair loss.

Questions:

> *What is currently putting me under pressure emotionally?*
> *What level of performance is expected in my situation?*
> *What is giving me such emotional stress?*
> *Early onset baldness: I look at my home with my parents.*
> *High achievement was expected; I grew up with it and consider it normal. I have assimilated the internalised expectations of high performance of my parents or my environment.*

Headache/migraine

Our head is our consciousness, a sort of authority that leads and controls us. It is precisely this control that attacks us through a headache. Headache, and even more so, migraine are self-attacks. They appear when we devalue ourselves and consequently we punish ourselves, for we have failed within our value system. People, who suffer frequently and violently from headaches and migraine, live in a value system that demands very high standards and they enslave themselves and others to these values. They are very critical of others and themselves. Whenever they do not attain the high expectations they have set themselves, their self-criticism expresses itself in headaches. The cause is always a critical judgement of failure. *"I was not good enough again! I do not love him/her enough; I am a rotten wife, or mother or daughter....so I am bad! I didn't try hard enough and I couldn't even reach my own goals..."* People suffering from headaches and migraine have internalised a negative belief pattern saying: *"I am no good... I am useless...I have failed...I*

51

deserve to be punished!" If children already have migraines, the parents should definitely examine their expectations honestly and stop imposing them on the children.

You can cure your own migraine with new, positive affirmations and by abandoning your very narrow and demanding value system.

Questions: (ask these whenever the pain starts)

> *What am I criticising about myself just now?*
> *Where do I think I have failed again, not done enough, been bad or not good enough?*
> *What am I punishing myself for this time?*
> *What value system am I applying with which to judge myself?*
> *What positive thoughts do I need to rid myself of these constraints?*

Heart

A heart condition signifies that we do not love our self enough. All cultures regard the heart as a symbol of love. However, contrary to what might be expected, it is not because others do not love us enough (in which case our lungs or kidneys would be affected), but it is because we do not love ourselves enough. People who suffer or even die from a heart attack have internalised a very strong belief, saying : *"I am not good enough! I am bad!"* Such people cannot achieve the very high level of achievement they have set themselves (as perfectionists) and so they punish themselves with a heart attack. During their whole life, they have been trying to prove to themselves and their environment that their negative belief system was wrong by constantly performing to the highest standards, so in the end their body is exhausted. As a rule, such people have overtaxed themselves during their entire life. They also find it very difficult to accept their own emotions, in particular aggression.

Questions:

> *What can I do to learn to love myself?*
> *Can I not simply accept the love of others for me?*
> *It is now high time to let go of the negative beliefs about myself: what positive experiences do I need now?*

Is it so important to me to be appreciated by others that I have made my self-esteem so very dependent on their judgment?

Hypochondria

People, who believe they are ill or are particularly afraid of serious illnesses, develop this anxiety to compensate for an unconscious wish to leave life via such an illness. Hypochondriacs feel weary of life and unable to cope with its challenges. They play unconsciously with the option of giving up totally on life through a fatal disease or at least partially through bringing on a grave illness which would at least permit them to step away from a permanent situation that they perceive as being too demanding or challenging.

Intestines

The intestines become diseased if we are afraid, but have to let go without wanting to. The intestines are both physically and symbolically the organ of "letting go." A considerable part of our fears are situated in the intestines, hence we talk about "being shit-scared!"

- Diarrhoea is always based on fear. Nearly everybody has experienced this just before an exam. Chronic diarrhoea signals a chronic fear. Of what?
- Constipation is a reaction to a desire not to let go. It means:"No! I want to keep him or her. I refuse to let go1" It often refers to ties that are difficult to break: children who leave home; separations and divorce; death etc. It might also concern material things that the person in question holds particularly dear and refuses to relinquish.
- Bowel cancer is almost always a physical reaction to a loss that cannot be worked through or "digested": death, divorce, children leaving home, grandchild moving etc - in other words, a separation in a close relationship.

Questions:

When exactly did the disorder start? What happened before then?

Intestinal bleeding: What is my gut crying about? What loss causes me such great sorrow? Who has hurt me so deeply through his departure or rejection?
Diarrhoea: What is currently terrifying me so much?
Constipation: Who or what do I want to hold on to although their loss seems inevitable?
Bowel cancer: What loss can I not come to terms with? Whom am I so attached to that I would rather die myself? What grief over the loss of an attachment is eating me up inside?

Joints

Joints suffer (rheumatism, arthritis or similar complaints) if we resist change in our thinking or our mental orientation. Symbolically, our joints are responsible for changes in direction, just as they are physically. If we refuse to change direction in our ideas or thoughts, either because we are obstinate or fearsome, then the joints are affected and the pain makes us feel our internal resistance.
Questions:

What change is being imposed on me by my life or by other people?
What anxiety is making it so difficult for me to alter my orientation in life, although it would be better for me?
Do I wish to continue to fight my own changes stubbornly and cripple myself in the process?
Looking at my life honestly, do I really feel that it is so bad that I need to fight change so strenuously?
Is there nothing positive to be gained by altering my views and my beliefs?

Kidneys

We have a right kidney and a left kidney which symbolise you and me. The kidneys represent our relationships and they fall ill if we feel hurt, neglected or unloved in our closest relationships (father, mother, partner, children, and close friends). The cause is always a very specific bond, in other words a single real person who has hurt

us. Conversely, we ourselves may have hurt a person who is very dear to us, in which case the kidneys might likewise react by ailing.
Questions:
> *What close person makes me feel that I have been hurt, neglected or unloved?*
> *Have I hurt a person who is very dear to me?*

Knees

Our knees become affected by feelings of humiliation or disadvantage. In a wider sense, knee complaints are an expression of mental obstinacy. We refuse to change even though other people or our circumstances demand it of us. In a manner of speaking, our ego resides in our knees shouting defiantly: "No! I won't give in!" People suffering from knee problems almost always consider giving in to be admitting to being inferior, or being defeated and even humiliated. Knee conditions are based on an unconscious thought pattern: the subject always thinks and feels in hierarchical terms. The world is divided from top to bottom; there are winners and losers, victory and defeat.

In all cultures, it is easy to understand the meaning of the knees. Kneeling is a universal gesture of humility, be it in prayer or before the authority of a king, guru or pope. Falling to one's knees before another person is to be humble and inferior (I below – you above) and shows one's respect for the other (your worth is greater than mine). A sore knee indicates a difficulty with giving in, accepting inferiority and not being in the right. Left knee: look at your relationship with your partner/ your mother. Right knee: look at your work, your conscious decisions, and your relationship with your father.

Questions:
> *Who or what makes me feel forced to give in or change?*
> *On what point do I feel I am definitely right?*
> *What change is making me particularly want to dig my heels in?*

Legs

Legs mean moving forwards in life.

Our left leg stands for our relationship with our mother, the right leg with our father. The section from our foot to our knee represents the first 7 years of age: the left the years with our mother, the right with our father. The section from the knee to the hip bone are symbolised by the following 7 years, viz. to 14 years of age.

A chronic problem with the leg (excepting the knee), such as phlebitis, open sores, tumour, skin irritations always at the same spot, etc. indicates a psychological injury in childhood that has not been overcome. According to where the damage is situated, we can discover when the bad experience happened. If the left leg is injured, the negative experience was connected with the mother, and if it was the right leg it would mean that it was connected with the father or a paternal figure.

Leg problems in general imply that we are reluctant to go forwards in life. An internal problem is holding us back. It might be an old problem, in which case the affliction is mostly chronic, or a current problem, which would then most probably be the result of an accident.

If the left leg is damaged, we might find it generally difficult to go forwards in our own close relationships, to build on them and develop them.

If the right leg is damaged, we might find it difficult to go forward in our work place or to build on and develop a conscious decision we made earlier.

Liver

Rage, aggression, hate, resentment and anger make the liver sick if these sentiments are repressed. A disorder of the liver is always associated with suppressed aggression. As a rule, people who cannot admit to their aggression tend to have liver trouble.

Question:

> *What made me so angry?*
> *Who made me so cross?*
> *What thought patterns stop me from admitting my*

aggressions?
Do I always need to be the "good guy" to myself and to
others? Why?
Do I believe that feelings are negative?

Lungs

The lungs represent our entire relationship with life itself. Our lungs are "the breath of life"; breathing in and breathing out is the most fundamental movement of life. The lungs fall ill if life no longer seems worth living, or if a very enveloping unhappiness about everything in life overcomes us.

Pneumonia is an alarm signal that our life nerve has been attacked and that some situation has arisen that encompasses everything and not just a part of our life. Our life nerve and our will to live are at stake. It is as though our will to live is located in our lungs. This organ is directly dependent on the LOVE in our life. If love has gone from our life, it becomes empty and senseless. That is the message of lungs that are afflicted: without love, life is pointless. The lungs tell us about primordial love and the most primitive sense of feeling safe and cosseted. If this is lacking, the lungs will always be an ailing organ. The lungs are connected with our earliest sense of confidence given to us by our mother. If the lungs become inflamed something really drastic needs to be done in order to reinvigorate and restore a person's will to live. A change is essential and an honest re-assessment of life is required. A first step is to look at the most important relationships. Experiencing love can redeem an ailing chest because it is through love that life regains a purpose. A person who is suffering from a serious disorder of the lungs needs to try again consciously to pull his life together, to say yes consciously to the innermost aspects of his personality and whole-heartedly to accept his own life in this world. When a person suffers a chronic lung disease, it means that he refuses to participate totally in his earthly existence and holds himself slightly aloof from the here and now, preferring to keep one leg in a sort of fanciful "other world", which rapidly leads to physical death. It is because the lungs reflect this basic attitude that lung cancer is often fatal. When the lungs are diseased the death wish becomes active.

Questions:

> *What is making my life pointless at the moment?*
> *Do I have love in my life?*
> *What exactly is attacking my will to live?*
> *Why do I want to give up and leave? Why do I not want to stay?*
> *What could give me a purpose again and motivate me to stay?*

Migraine (see headache)
Significance: self-criticism, self punishment

Multiple sclerosis
This illness is the body's reaction to a serious feeling of being a victim. The sufferer will have been very deeply hurt and disappointed by a close person (generally a partner) and is now reacting defiantly over having been exploited. The psychological mechanics work unconsciously in the following way: "Now look at what you have done to me! You have made me terribly ill! It is your fault that I feel so sick!" The creeping progression of the paralysis in the body shows the extent of the enormous feeling of being a victim. Unconsciously the blame for the affliction is heaped on the other person.
Questions:

> *Who has hurt me and disappointed me so deeply?*
> *I am conscious of my feelings of being the victim; should they really rule me?*

Neck
Obstinacy makes one's neck rigid and painful. A flexible neck symbolises our capacity to perceive other perspectives. We speak of a "stiff-necked" person to say he is self-willed because his stubbornness actually manifests itself in the neck. If we are inflexible and stick determinedly to our own views refusing to see any other reasonable angle, our neck will suffer. Neck problems are almost

always an opposition to outside pressure to accept a new perspective and give up some old attitudes. I see this a lot in my seminars: certain people almost always suffer from neck problems during my seminars!

Questions:

> *What new views am I rejecting at the moment?*
> *Why do I hold on to my own views so stubbornly?*
> *Why do new ideas make me so easily insecure and angry?*

Neurodermatitis (see skin)

This complaint is a bodily reaction to an emotional injury that the sufferer does not wish consciously to recognise and he therefore represses it into his body. A person who is very close to me and who has emotional power over me has hurt me, rejected me or not accepted me (almost always a parent or both parents).

Nose

The nose stands for self-knowledge. If we have a problem with our nose or if it is injured, we are fighting some understanding of our self that is due to be dealt with and we should face the problem openly and frankly.

Nose bleed: Grief about oneself. I am crying about myself.

Cold: Dissatisfaction with my present situation.

Runny nose: Sadness, repressed weeping

Sinusitis: Aggression against a close person

Obsessional neurosis

This psychological illness is based on an internal conviction – I call it a set of beliefs or a belief pattern- that says:*"I am bad! I am unclean! I do everything wrong!"* In seriously bad cases, the belief pattern says: *"I have no right to exist! So I must do everything right and perform to the highest level in order to earn that right!"* For an obsessional person every little rule or habit becomes a question of "to be or not to be". A rule equals coercion, so complying with it to the letter means: *"I am allowed to be here provided I do everything* *right and only if I do not break any rules!"*To act against a rule means: *"I am bad, I am evil, I do everything wrong and I should not be here at all!"*An obsessional person does not only have an inferiority complex but he even questions his right to live. That is why he tries so hard to follow his obsessions because they give him a spurious sense of security. If he does things right he can, at least for the moment, earn himself some kind of justification for existing. In order to combat this illness I would always recommend psychotherapy because it is almost impossible to contend with this emotional dilemma on one's own.

Otitis: see ears

Pancreas (see diabetes)

Prostate
This organ symbolises the male principle. The prostate falls ill if a man rejects or no longer values his masculinity. Most men who suffer from the prostate have a strong need for acknowledgement. A man tends to define his own masculinity in specific terms of acknowledgement which are mostly determined by his level of success in his profession. A prostate problem is based on a man's own very rigid and narrow image of masculinity. If he loses his job, and with it a particular form of success expressing his masculinity, a man develops a deep sense of worthlessness and failure. Many men will have spent their lives aimed almost exclusively at achieving professional success. Then they are suddenly at home without any real duties and worse still, without the old structures for achievement, so that their self-esteem as a man collapses. A man in this situation may feel that he has forfeited his own masculinity. Prostate cancer is a self-aggression according to the motto: "I have failed utterly as a man; therefore I deserve to die for my failure!"
Unemployment and lack of success are not always the reason for disease. Partnerships too can cause a man to feel inadequate and lead

to prostate disease. However the root always lies in a diminished sense of self-value and doubts about his worth as a male.

Questions:

When exactly did the physical problem appear?

What withdrawal of masculine acknowledgement preceded this affliction?

In what way do I not feel like a full-blooded male in my partnership?

Rheumatism

This ailment crops up when self-conscious people cannot assert themselves and consequently attach themselves to a victim situation. Their aggressive energy builds up within the body, generally in the joints that stand for changes in direction, and this energy manifests itself as rheumatism. The sufferer feels unconsciously that he is dominated by others and although he resents this, he refuses to admit it because he would then have to react consciously. The emotional energy that causes rheumatism is a mixture of wanting to avoid conflict and yet holding on obstinately to inhibited behaviour. The sufferer feels victimised, he feels subjugated and controlled by other people, and his rheumatism will finally make it manifestly clear that he is also physically a victim.

Questions:

Who do I think dominates and subjugates me?

Why do I give other people so much power over me?

What fears deter me from pushing through my own wishes?

What do I really want?

What set of beliefs about myself limit me so much?

When will I finally start insisting that my own wishes are carried out?

Do I really want to let my inhibitions hold me back so much in future?

Respiratory system.
Air is the "breath of life" (see also "Lungs"). If the organs that provide us with air are afflicted, our whole life is seriously disturbed. Having breathing difficulties can very quickly become life threatening. Symbolically, it means that we are not getting enough out of life, life is passing us by. Our problem may well have started due to outside factors, but it has now affected our own basic frame of mind. These feelings have begun to make our life so hard: we feel needy and lacking in loving affection, we yearn to feel safe and wrapped in emotional warmth

Scalp (see also hair)
Our scalp suffers if we are under emotional pressure or stress. Dandruff, excema and other skin irritations on the scalp are produced when we feel pushed about by external factors, such as high demands (which lead to hair loss) or stress in love or partnerships etc.

Schizophrenia
This mental illness is the expression of a very serious psychological negation of communal living and interaction with other people. Schizophrenia is a radical retreat into another world and thus a resounding "No!" to the world that we share with other people. Schizophrenics live in a state of tension with existence, in that they do not really want to be here, not in this life and not with these people. Schizophrenia enables them to dissociate themselves from the consensus that society has created based on the way we see and interpret reality. A precondition for a person to "create" schizophrenia is a very sensitive nature and a basic sense of being lost in this world. In fact, before he was afflicted by this mental illness, he would never really have been of this world nor adjusted to this life. As a rule, we find that there has been some trauma in infancy relating to mother bonding: lack of warmth, love and safety. The illness gives the sufferer a way of dealing with this conflict: staying here but without being here in a social sense. He creates a world of his own, separate from the world of others. This kind of person sometimes lets spirits help him and gives them a home. In this

case external spiritual beings take possession of him in the truest sense of the word. These spirits generally exacerbate the sufferer's problems but they also give him access to extraordinary perceptions. (cf. Acts of healing by Jesus in the New Testament, half of which were exorcising evil spirits) These external spirits sometimes take complete control of the person, for instance through voices giving commands that almost exclusively aim at destructive actions. Such spirits park themselves in the aggressions of the host, settling into his opposition and negation of the world around him. Traditional medicine has no chance of getting rid of these beings, so that spiritual help is needed. In such cases, it is very important to take these voices seriously and not to dismiss them as hallucinations.
Questions:

When exactly did the illness begin?
Was there a trigger, and if so, what was it?
Do I wish to continue to live in the shadows?
Am I ready to exorcise these spirits from my personality?

Sexual organs

The significance of our sexual organs does not actually need any explanation: they stand for our male or female sexuality and any problems connected with that. If you experience physical difficulties in this area, you should definitely take an honest look at your sex life. Often, dissatisfaction with your partner or an earlier bad experience, such as abuse, may play a part. A negative mindset can also influence one's sexual organs, like thinking: "I am no good in bed! I never reach orgasm, so I am a failure!" etc.

Sexual diseases

I believe that the spiritual cause for sexual disease is a feeling of guilt or "sexual impurity". The disease is a punishment for unconscious guilt feelings connected with one's own sexuality. Self-healing through meditation should focus on the whole area of partnerships to discover the unconscious sense of guilt or a whole slew of negative beliefs about one's own value as a sexual partner.
Questions:

What unconscious set of beliefs do you have as a sexual

63

partner?
What guilt feeling is bothering you in this area?
What are you punishing yourself for with this disease?

Shoulders

Shoulder disorders occur basically when we cannot or will not support current experiences. We have "overloaded" ourselves or life has done this with our help. If the left shoulder is affected, the overload is related to an experience with our partner or other relationship (for example separation, conflicts, worry and stress over the children, excessive demands, and worries over parents...)

If the right shoulder is affected, the overload relates to an experience in the work place and is connected to some conscious decisions we have made (for example excessive demands at work, new job, conflicts at work...)

Tensed up shoulders mean that the individual is under a great deal of pressure and stress. He cannot "loosen up".

Skin

The skin is our tactile organ, which suffers if we feel spiritually hurt by others but refuse consciously to acknowledge this wound.

- The main disorder in this context is **neurodermatitis,** which mostly affects children. Its background is a psychological wound inflicted by one or other parent. The child feels insufficiently loved and cosseted and needs a greater sense of being emotionally protected.
  Babies who can already feel within their mother's womb that they are not really wanted or that they are insufficiently loved and accepted are now-a-days often even born with neuro-dermatitis.
- **Psoriasis** is the result of a long lasting emotional problem with another person or group. It is a "skin stress" reflecting the internal emotional stress.
- **Dandruff** is like a kind of carapace protecting us from stress and any possible attacks by others.

64

Sleep disorders

Sleep disorders are a result of fear or loss of control. Sleep is like a kind of death or faint which switches off our waking consciousness and lets the unconscious step in. It is generally only in sleep that we meet up in our dreams with our unconscious and our repressed worries lodged there. A sleep disorder means that we fear our own unconscious mind. Why? Because a great deal is happening there and massive emotions and problems are pushing to come to the surface. To stop this from happening, we stop sleeping. Our head simply will not give in: As the controller, it remains alert in order that supposed safety is assured. The emotional problem surging forward from the unconscious is perceived as a great danger. Disturbed sleep is an attempt to contain the danger and our fear.
Questions:

What is trying to push out from the depths of my soul into my awareness?
What is making me so terribly afraid?
Why do I not trust my internal wisdom?
Who could help me now to find a way to understand my problem?

Slipped disc

The discs and the whole lower back can be affected if we find ourselves in an emotional state of stress and existentialist "angst". Stress, brought on by excessive demands, leads to the following thought process: "This is too much! I can't cope! I shall fail and then I shall lose all my confidence!" The perceived feeling of being overburdened by too many tasks, challenges and worries compresses the vertebrae. The additional fear of failure can heighten into an existentialist angst ("If I fail, I will lose my job, my partner, my children etc."). This massive mixture of feeling over-taxed and being out of control and thus losing everything including one's safety net, is frequently the cause of lower back problems.
Questions:

When exactly did the symptoms start?
What tasks or challenges did I face at that time?
What stressed me out then?

65

*What basic tenet or doctrine do I believe in, that might
cause this fear of failure?*

Spleen

This organ becomes unwell if we are beset by dark spiritual forces. It reacts against spirits that are attempting to intrude on us and possess us. The spleen gives us a warning by ailing even when we simply encounter other people who are possessed (see epilepsy and schizophrenia). In a way, the spleen acts as a "red warning light" for the body.
Questions:

*When exactly did the spleen become unwell?
Who did I meet who could possibly be associated with dark
forces?
Have I taken part in a spiritual seminar or in a ceremony?
Have I been watching horror or pornographic films?
Is there anyone in my environment who seems menacing or
spooky to me?*

Stomach

The stomach suffers illness if we cannot "digest" an experience, a situation or a great misfortune. We have swallowed our feelings and we cannot "stomach" them. Our stomach will also tend to revolt if we are stressed out.
Questions:

*What experience do I find so hard to digest?
What exactly is upsetting my stomach?
What causes me to feel stressed or under emotional
pressure?*

Teeth

Teeth problems occur when we find it difficult to make decisions. Either we would like to make a decision but are too diffident or we have actually made a decision and are now having second thoughts and worries. We might also be thinking that we ought to make a decision but we are pushing this thought away. Teeth troubles always reflect an internal, as yet unconscious conflict connected with decision making. Here again, it is worth taking a closer look: left side – the conflict is probably in connection with partnership or relationships. Right side: the conflict is probably in connection with work and our actions within a wider circle of our world.

Throat

The whole area of the throat symbolises our self-expression, and hence many of the needs that might be called egoistic. Our aggressiveness, our troubles, and wounding or disparaging words "stick in our throat" because we are afraid that we might be punished or rejected if we utter them. The area of the throat is afflicted if we are reluctant to express our annoyance, unease or self-centred desires.

Tinnitus (see ears)

Toes

Our toes have the same symbolic meaning as our fingers (see above), but they also indicate a more fundamental problem that has to do with our standing in life. In my experience toe problems are often associated with the parental relationship (left foot mother, right foot father).

Tongue

There are many sayings that give us hints about the symbolic significance of the tongue. "I bit my tongue" (I didn't say what I desperately wanted to say); "It was on the tip of my tongue" (I

67

wanted to say something but could not express the thought or find the right words); someone speaks with a "forked tongue" (insincere, with double meaning, sly).

The tongue becomes affected if words cannot be spoken that urgently need to be formulated: above all, angry words, aggressive words and words to make demands for one's own needs.

Cancer of the tongue seems to occur more frequently these days and it shows us that words are repressed into the unconscious whereas they urgently need to be SPOKEN.

Questions:

> *What angry or aggressive words are you holding back?*
> *Who are these words directed at?*
> *Why is it so difficult for you to stand up for yourself?*
> *With whose tongue are you speaking and why?*

Vomiting

There is something in my current situation that makes me want to "vomit". I should look carefully what my problem is. It lies in the immediate present.

Warts

Warts symbolise the saying of a "thorn in the flesh". Warts are the expression of aggression and vexation. Something or someone is getting on my nerves. As warts normally occur on hands or feet, their specific meaning will be found according to which fingers or toes are affected. A special feature of warts is that it is not enough to dig up the problem from the unconscious and lift it into the conscious, but it is also necessary to change things externally in life to get rid of the warts.

Womb – the maternal principle

Health problems to do with the womb are in my experience caused by maternal feelings of guilt towards one's own children. Cancer of the womb is a dramatic guilt complex, often associated with an abortion but at least connected with a notion of failing one's children

68

as a mother. "As a mother, I am very much at fault". "I deserve to die" (cancer cases). Cancer of the womb is a massive self-punishment. A woman sentences herself unconsciously to atone for her own faults. Even if there is no such dramatic intrusion as an abortion to cause the womb to be afflicted, she nevertheless has a sense that she has not given the child enough or not loved him enough. Even women who have never had babies can judge themselves on that very count and condemn themselves because their mother or other close friends and family expected them to give birth, and they now see themselves as failures and incomplete women. In order to heal such cases, it is absolutely necessary to make these feelings of failure and guilt surface into the conscious mind and to work through them there. In cancer cases psychotherapy is highly recommended to support the sufferer.

Question:

> *Where do I feel that I have failed as a mother?*
> *Why am I assailed by feelings of guilt?*
> *Which steps or decisions have I taken to cause this guilt?*
> *Was there an abortion? Was my child given away for adoption? Did I turn away from my child?*
> *Was there one of my children whom I could not really accept?*
> *What can I do to forgive myself?*
> *If there have never been any children: Do I blame myself for that? Does that detract from my value as a woman?*

Suggested methods for healing one self

When exactly did the illness start?

Try to find the exact time of the onset of the disease, or in other words, when you noticed the symptoms. The body generally needs a little time to transform the feelings and problems that have been repressed into the unconscious and to make them materialise into a noticeable ailment.

Only accidents have their cause in the immediate present. Many illnesses have an internal spiritual cause long before the onset of symptoms. If you are able to determine fairly precisely when the disorder started, go back a bit before that time and ask yourself the following questions:

*What was happening in my life during the time before the
onset of the ailment?*
What experiences did I have in that period?
What influences was I exposed to?
What changes have taken place in my life?

Remember: as you are dealing with a problem that you are not yet conscious of, it can take some time before you become aware of any connection between an event in your life and the onset of your illness. Check out everything that you can think of, even if at first you can see no possible connection between the event or experience and your illness.

What exactly is the illness doing to me?

Now you should note as clearly as possible what the disease is doing to you. This is not a matter of abstract analysis but really simple descriptions, such as: You cannot walk anymore, you cannot stand up straight, you cannot eat certain foods, you cannot hear, taste, or see as well anymore...
Now ask the following questions:

What exactly does the disease prevent me from doing?

Which organ exactly is affected?
What does the disease force me to do (am I obliged to do things I would not normally have to do?)
What must I possibly avoid (e.g. in case of allergy)?

What exactly does the illness give you?

Every illness has a positive side effect – if we look closely and honestly. Even a fatal illness has an effect in that it allows death to resolve a conflict and to end a depressing situation in life. So your illness is somehow also a way of getting something that you believed that you were otherwise unable to attain (e.g. rest, relaxation, cosseting by others, attention, an excuse not to have to continue as before etc.) Ask yourself the following questions:
What exactly does the illness allow me to have or do?
What unconscious need is fulfilled by means of my illness?
In what way does my incapacity satisfy my need (e.g. I cannot hear well, because people irritate me with their blabbering... I have to lie down: finally I can get some rest and let others worry...)?
Why do I feel that I can only satisfy this need by having this illness? Check your set of beliefs!

What exactly is your real problem?

In this decisive phase of your honest analysis, you can discover through the pattern of your illness what your, as yet unconscious, problem is and how it is causing your ailment at an energy level. The better you recognise your own problem, the faster your body will heal. No taboos! You must now be totally honest with yourself!
You will find your clues by looking at the symbolic significance of the ailing organ. Once you have recognised and accepted what the organ or disorder stands for unconsciously, you can track down your actual problem. **You should describe the problem carefully and clearly,** e.g. nut allergy: I have a problem with male sexuality. Or

diarrhoea: I am afraid. Or knee problems: I will not give in, I feel humiliated...

The energy contained in your problem is emotion. Make yourself find some of the following feelings and try to experience them consciously:

>**Feelings of guilt**. Note: unconscious guilt feelings are always followed by self-punishment!
>
>**Feelings of failure.**
>
>**Feelings of shame** (especially for blame and failure).
>
>**Aggressions:** hate, rage, resentment, anger, vengeance!
>
>**Feelings of being victimised** – they also unconsciously produce aggressions!
>
>**Fears** – e.g. fear of loss; existential angst; fear of failure; fear of abandonment; fear of loneliness, of devotion, of change...etc.
>
>**Barriers:** obstinacy, perfectionism, ambition, refusals (e.g. refusing to grow up) and emotional resistance to development, honesty and clarity.
>
>**Negative belief patterns about yourself:** every disease – yes, every single disease - and all connected problems and repressed feelings are based on negative thoughts about yourself. You believe some negative rubbish like for instance:"I am bad, I am not lovable, I am feeble, a failure, I am to blame, I deserve to be punished, life is rotten and unfair; I am always the one to cop it; nobody loves me; I am a loser; I shouldn't be here at all...etc."

These feeling must be drawn out into the open, consciously, and thus be allowed to flow away from the unconscious. Remember that the energy of these feelings is responsible for your disease. **Healing is achieved by discharging the burden of these emotional energies from your body by making these feelings rise into your conscious and experiencing them consciously in your mind.** Many of these repressed feelings need a lot of time to flow away and to be processed in the conscious mind. You might need professional help through a psychologist or other counsellor to be successful. It is worth your while and you should get yourself this sort of support!

What decisions and changes are required to return to good health?

You have now found out what the real problem is that causes you a physiological disorder.

Step one:
Now the repressed feelings must be allowed to flow into your conscious. It is not enough to simply acknowledge the problem intellectually. This would not be sufficient to regain your health because the energy with which you made your body sicken is the power of the feelings that you refused so far to feel. The repressed feelings must be perceived consciously so that they may finally depart. You have to consciously feel your fear, anger, helplessness, disappointment, grief etc. This is disagreeable, so we fall ill, because it seems easier to us to endure the disease rather than to face these nasty feelings. In this phase, it often makes sense to get yourself some help such as through a good psychotherapist, through your church or other spiritual guidance or through a friend. Face up to your repressed feelings!

Step two:
Change is required. The magnitude of change will depend on your problem. There is no healing without change. Many people prefer to die rather than to change themselves and their situation. Fear of change is enormous and one of the most massive causes of repression.
In every case - in every single case without exception – you will have to change your set of beliefs (your innermost attitudes and convictions), your negative thoughts about yourself, your environment, life... You have been stuck too long in a situation that was so not right for you. Your disease is a cry for change – for life, for healing. Some diseases demand really big changes of you, such as giving up your work, ending a partnership, leaving certain people who are very close to you, moving house etc.

73

By now, having clarified your true problem and called up your repressed feelings into your conscious and having taken a clear decision about positive changes, you will have started to note the first signs of healing in your body. Promise!

Note: in any case decisions are always necessary. If you have a disease that threatens your life, it is always imperative that you should make a new decision in favour of life. This decision has to operate right down into your subconscious and be emotionally grounded. Straightforward cerebral decisions are not sufficient to bring about healing.

Honesty instead of fighting the illness!

I hear again and again people say they are *"fighting their illness."* That means that all their energy is spent in repression. Illness is not an enemy that we have to fight against! It is a part of us, an expression of a pressing problem that wishes to be recognised and accepted by our conscious. A fight against an illness is a fight against oneself. You would do better to invest your energy in life, in clarification and healing. Whenever we fight *"against"* something, we are actually reinforcing what we are fighting against.
I would recommend that you should stop fighting your disease because you are actually using up your energy in reinforcing your repression.

Be honest! Listen to yourself! Pay attention to yourself, listen also to the words you say. Listen to your illness; learn the language of your body!

Healing and guilt

In order to heal your body you may have to pay a price, because you will have to take certain decisions that may cause you to feel guilty within your set of beliefs. The stronger and more threatening the disease, the more urgent and imperative the call for change will be. You have fallen ill because you are afraid of change. This fear has many aspects and one of them is guilt. You do not want to feel guilty about other people, so you shy away from abandoning them or demanding that they take your needs on board and that they will have to face up to the consequences of your changes.

To cure ourselves we often have to offend against the expectations of people who are close to us, such as our parents, partners, children, friends, colleagues and bosses. We often have to contravene value judgements of other people and be seen by them as "bad", "egoistic" or even "evil" in order to regain our health. And most of all, we might well need to violate our own sense of morality and our value judgements which will of course make us feel bad.

Life itself imposes guilt on us. No life exists in innocence because guilt is a basic given of life and an incontrovertible necessity. Just remember, however, that you can choose who you should feel guilty about. If you cannot bear to wrong other people, you will come to wrong yourself. Disease is already a physiological expression of an existing imbalance within yourself. It is imperative in many cases, but in particular in very serious illnesses, to make far-reaching transformations, like leaving one's family, moving house, starting up a new business, deserting false friends, deliberately turning one's back on parental expectations, disappointing other people or perhaps airing existing disagreements and thus causing others to feel discomfort, anger, hate, disappointment, misapprehension and other such emotions.

The healing process demands that you should definitely detach yourself from an excessively moral understanding of guilt or blame. Try to regard guilt more philosophically or spiritually as a necessary "greasing agent" or "catalyst" to become involved in life. Guilt feelings involve us in our world and make us slip further into the act of living. The conflicts they engender enhance our self-knowledge and increase our learning. Attempting to avoid blame is like trying to avoid living.

Let me give you a morally neutral definition of guilt: *being the cause of an imbalance*. We never, ever, can hold everything in perfect balance. So we must be to blame. So I accept that. When you are sick, you have already pushed yourself off balance. To cure yourself, you often have to push other people off their balance (and they may only seem to be in balance anyway). You are not doing this on purpose, but because the change you need may generate that kind of imbalance in your network of relationships. If you avoid taking the blame and feeling guilty, you will become even more ill. Do not feel afraid of being guilty, just admit the blame consciously. Feel it, accept it. It is part of the healing process. But don't succumb to it! Do not let guilt feelings stop you from making the decisions that are necessary for your cure. Decide! Act! Accept guilt feelings!

Conclusion

Disease originates in us through taboos. We are afraid to take cognizance of a problem, or certain conflicts and feelings. That is normal. These fears and the resulting repressions are part of our human existence.

To be honest with oneself is a difficult task. We find it is easier to be critical, which is always a negative value judgement. Everybody finds it easy to criticise and hence to devalue himself even if this often happens unconsciously.

Total honesty can only be achieved against a background of self-acceptance. If you want to work successfully with the information presented here, you must first learn to accept yourself as you are, with all your emotions, problems and conflicts. Self-acceptance is the precondition for regaining your health. In order to achieve this curative self-acceptance, you must abandon your old value judgements about right and wrong. Deep in your unconscious you have learnt to rate yourself and other people according to the values of your parents and other persons in authority.

Make yourself aware of these value judgements and let them slowly float away. I shall give you other criteria for *"right"* and *"wrong"*: Try instead "good" and "bad" and define both as follows:

"Good" is everything that serves life, liveliness and growth.

"Bad" is everything that hinders or even prevents life, liveliness and growth. In this value system, illness is "good" because it helps you to strengthen your liveliness by recognising your blockages and overcoming them. Your awareness will become wider and deeper. Everything you discover about yourself is "good" because it serves your life, your liveliness and your growth. And everything that supports you on the way to this recognition is also good. You, yourself are good, because you are here, because you are alive, because you were created to live, to grow and to gain insight.

If you consult this booklet frequently and work on yourself, at some point you will realise that there is basically only one truly big and deep-seated problem for everyone: **A lack of self-esteem.**

All the other problems and conflicts that we encounter with ourselves and life are generated by our lack of self-esteem. Disease, too, originates from this fundamental problem. All the repressed problems, conflicts and feelings that are the cause of disease serve to confirm our sense of worthlessness – which is in fact the reason for repression in the first place. We believe that we would really be bad, not good enough, stupid or inadequate if we admitted these feelings. But that is all rubbish. These are only negative thoughts that we took on board when we were children. These thoughts do not correspond to any reality except that which we have created for ourselves.

Please make it clear to yourself that we human beings have not and cannot ascribe a value to ourselves. Our value was given to us with our existence. It comes from our Creator, and only from Him. Even our parents cannot give us nor take from us our value. And yet, their feelings toward us mould our sense of self-esteem. But remember that our feelings about our self-worth are only feelings and do not have any reality. You are valuable, quite independently from what you are doing or have done. Our value has nothing to do with our actions. Nor does it depend in any way on our thoughts and feelings. Our value is a fixed, *objective* quantity. I never use the term *"objective"* otherwise because basically we humans are never

77

objective and never can be. However, this value that was given to us with our existence is not human but holy and divine and so, exceptionally, I feel justified in using this normally non-applicable term.

I close with this final note reminding you of your incontrovertible value as a being of the universe, a being created by a power that far exceeds our imagination and whose love surpasses every sensation that we can ever possibly feel. I hope that the knowledge that I have shared with you here has been able to help you with your healing and your knowledge and that it will continue to be helpful to you in future. Everything will turn out alright. Even if some things take a little time. Be confident!

Klaus Koeppe

Contact: e-mail: nakodaman@web.de